AF273415

MADELYN LAKE

TIME FOR BED

The Essential Guide to Enjoying Quality Sleep, Learn Proven Methods to Hack Your Sleep to Finally Sleep Soundly and Peacefully at Night

Descrierea CIP a Bibliotecii Naţionale a României
MADELYN LAKE
  TIME FOR BED. The Essential Guide to Enjoying Quality Sleep, Learn Proven Methods to Hack Your Sleep to Finally Sleep Soundly and Peacefully at Night / Madelyn Lake – Bucharest: Editura My Ebook, 2021
  ISBN

MADELYN LAKE

TIME FOR BED

The Essential Guide to Enjoying Quality Sleep, Learn Proven Methods to Hack Your Sleep to Finally Sleep Soundly and Peacefully at Night

My Ebook Publishing House
Bucharest, 2021

TABLE OF CONTENTS

INTRODUCTION

Sleep is the golden chain that ties health and our bodies together.

Thomas Dekker

Every one of us suffers from insomnia at some point in our lives. It could be triggered by stressful periods in our careers, a personal crisis, fear of an upcoming event or worrying about finances may keep us awake and restless. Feelings of guilt or grief are another culprit.

Whatever the reasons that keep you tossing and turning, you know how it feels to drag yourself out of bed in the morning. You are sapped of energy. Your body aches and your brain is foggy. You feel irritable and grumpy. Your sleepless night is going to reflect on your whole day – and not for the better.

Over time, sleep issues can become extremely debilitating. Persistent lack of sleep will negatively impact your career, social life, and personal relationships. At times, they may challenge your very sanity.

For some people, insomnia is a chronic issue. For others, it comes and goes sometimes. While for most people, insomnia may be closely related to the quality or length of sleeping hours. Sleep deprivation can really take its toll on our mind and physical health.

It can lead to serious issues such as depression, high blood pressure and an out of control hormone system. This puts our body at a higher risk of chronic illnesses and speeds up the aging process.

Since you are reading this book, you probably have a sleep problem and want to do something about it. You may have tried countless remedies (the warm glass of milk before bed or counting sheep). You may have resorted to prescription medication, adding to your problem the risk of addiction.

And yet, nothing seems to work. Are you then doomed to live with your sleep problems for the rest of your life? Absolutely not.

Biohacking is the solution to beating sleep deprivation issues once and for all. It's totally safe, easy, relatively cost-free and guaranteed to help you overcome stubborn sleep issues.

The biohacking tools you're about to discover will help you easily change and regulate your individual sleep patterns. They will help you tailor a plan that will result in concrete changes to optimize sleep, and improve your overall health and wellbeing.

Incorporating these biohacking techniques into your lifestyle will make the changes permanent so that you can always be assured of sound, restful sleep.

CHAPTER 1

BIOHACKING BRIEFLY EXPLAINED

Do you eat a lot of fatty fish to improve your brain health? Do you use essential oils to relieve stress and boost your mood? Perhaps you follow a diet high in antioxidants or work out regularly to improve your cardiovascular health. If that's the case, then you are already a biohacker! In fact, most of us are biohackers in some form or another without even knowing it.

What is Biohacking?

Biohacking is the process of making changes to your lifestyle habits in order to "hack" the body's biological functions and achieve positive health changes.

❑ Biohacking is simply "do-it-yourself" biology. Simple changes (such as in diet, exercise and sleep habits) are made to improve health, safeguard from disease and overcome issues like sleep deprivation.

❏ It is a fairly new practice and although it has its basis in biology, is not considered a science per se. However, its potentials could be huge. Studies on the field are ongoing and the findings are very promising. Biohacking has been already shown to have a major impact on many areas of physical and mental health.

❏ Biohacking is an experimental process because not all body cycles and rhythms are the same. Some people may respond to certain "hacks" while others will not. Therefore, it's a process of trying out different hacks to find out which one works best for you. This absolutely does not mean experimenting with your body in any way that can cause harm. The tools are perfectly safe to play around with and see which ones - if not all of them - improve your sleep.

❏ The main experts in the field of biohacking are Dave Asprey and Ben Greenfield. They experiment on themselves, develop new products and hacks in the field of nutrition and fitness and share them with the world.

There are three categories of biohacking:

1. **Nutrigenomics** is related to nutrition, stress management and hacking your surrounding environment, such as sound and light.

2. **DIYBIO** or do-it-yourself biology. This is where non-professional scientists conduct experiments in biohacking and share the results with likeminded people. The goal is to prove that the average laymen can become a successful biohacker.

3. **Grinder biohacking** focuses on technology such as implants and chemical supplements for hacking the body's biology. This is absolutely NOT recommended as the risks may be far greater than the benefits. This is better left to the total fanatics.

What should you focus on?

Sleep scientists tell us that it's not the number of hours that matter. It is the quality of your sleep that is essential for physical and mental health.

Many people sleep for 7 – 8 hours a night but still wake up feeling drained and unrested. This is because the quality of their sleep is poor. They are unable to enter into the state of deep sleep that relaxes and rejuvenates the body. Quality sleep means waking up energized and filled with vitality, regardless of how many hours you have slept. This needs to be your main focus; not just falling asleep, but sleeping well.

We can use a number of safe and natural biohacking techniques to improve our overall sleep quality. The following chapters will discuss some of the most popular and successful sleep hacks. These will help you:

- ❑ Overcome insomnia
- ❑ Fall asleep faster
- ❑ Improve the duration of sleep
- ❑ Improve the quality of sleep
- ❑ Promote deep, restful sleep

Some so-called experts claim that biohacking requires various gadgets and complex measurements to monitor brain waves and other responses. Honestly, this is completely unnecessary.

Always remember that nobody knows your body better than you. You will know what works best for you by how you feel. You will be able to measure the results by how much your sleep improves.

You may find that you enjoy biohacking so much that you want to delve deeper. As your knowledge and skill increases, you may want to try gadgets and measuring tools. But for now, let's keep things simple.

CHAPTER 2

BANISH BLUE LIGHT

Science tells us that light from the blue side of the spectrum disturbs the brain's production of melatonin, a hormone that regulates sleeping and waking. Exposure to blue light sources, especially in the evening, can drastically disturb your sleep.

Blue light can be light coming in through the window, as well as light from regular and LED bulbs. Digital screens including PCs, laptops, tablets, and TV screens are also huge emitter of blue light.

This hack is simple. Keeping all light out of your bedroom is the fastest and most effective ways to improve sleep.

There are several ways you can do this:

➢ **Use blackout curtains** to completely block out any daylight from filtering in. This is especially beneficial for late sleepers and people who work night shifts and sleep during the day.

➢ **A low-intensity amber night light** is fine if you absolutely cannot sleep in a totally dark room. These types of bulbs do not give off blue light. A good idea is to install dim amber lights in the hallway as well for those trips to the bathroom. This will help you quickly fall asleep again when you are back in bed.

➢ **Invest in a blue light-filtering sleep mask.** However, note that your whole body absorbs blue light through the skin. If this hack doesn't work for you, you will need to try the blackout curtains.

➢ **Ensure that your home lighting is sleep-friendly**. Our body starts producing melatonin a couple of hours before we go to bed, making us feel sleepy. However, too-bright lighting in the home, as well as television and computer screens, can inhibit the production of melatonin. Keep your home lighting dim (amber or red and yellow spectrum lighting is the best choice) - and don't watch TV or sit in front of the computer directly before going to bed.

This is because when your skin absorbs blue light, it starts producing cortisol, a hormone that increases alertness and weakens the effect of sleep-inducing melatonin.

➢ **Wear amber-tinted glasses** during the last 3-4 hours of daylight. This is another simple hack that supports "dim light melatonin production". This technical term means the production of melatonin during evening hours. Amber-tinted glasses are glasses that have yellow or orange lenses and are very inexpensive – but they could be just the hack you need for better sleep. They are available on Amazon in a variety of styles, as well as elsewhere online.

Become aware of the blue light sources surrounding you during the evening and banish them. This hack should give you fast results where you induce an improvement in your sleep in a few days.

CHAPTER 3

INVEST IN A SLEEP APP

Sleep apps are scientifically designed to give you a good night's sleep. They are easy to use and contain diverse features to choose from and experiment with, which is what we are recommended to do when biohacking.

They are crafted specifically to calm your brainwaves and create a relaxing experience that helps you drift into restful sleep. Optimally, it will help maintain restful sleep throughout the night.

Sleep apps typically give you a choice of audio recordings of soothing sounds that calm the brain and induce sleep. These include the sound of soft rain, ocean waves, wind rustling through trees and other nature sounds. Some apps offer guided meditation, white noise, and various ambient sounds.

Some apps also offer a wide range of relaxing classical and contemporary music so there's something for all tastes and preferences. It's fun to experiment with these different sounds and find the ones that best hack your sleep.

Other features include:

- Dashboards that display sleep patterns and percentage of quality sleep. Some apps can even measure snoring.

- If you are artistically inclined, apps like Recolor allow you to create brain-relaxing artwork. You are provided with a specific color palette designed to calm anxiety and promote sleep.

- A number of apps contain hypnosis tracks to calm and relax the brain.

- Some contain alarms to help you synchronize short naps during the day.

Popular apps on the market include Sleep Cycle, Pillow, Digipill, Recolor and Sleep Time. Most sleep apps are free for both android and iPhones. Those with more sophisticated features range from $3 to $9.99.

Helpful tip: White noise, in general, is a great sleep-inducer and numerous studies back this up. It keeps your brainwaves steady helps maintain sound asleep all night. If you choose not to use a sleep app, you can easily access white noise with a fan. A ceiling fan or a regular fan will work equally well. Simply keep it on all night. The sound will lull you to sleep and the consistent whirring will help sleep deeply throughout the night.

Try out a couple of the free apps ones first. If you enjoy using it and get good results, great! If not, you haven't needlessly wasted any money.

CHAPTER 4

SEEK OUT THE SUN

This is a case in which blue light from the sun can actually help us sleep better! Staying away from blue light in the evening is necessary as discussed in chapter 1. However, exposure to blue light during the daytime is another matter, so don't get confused.

Exposure to sunlight helps our body maintain its circadian rhythm by sending signals to our pituitary gland and hypothalamus. Circadian rhythm simply means our body's internal clock. Keeping it balanced and stable is essential for quality sleep. Our circadian rhythm also regulates a number of important hormones, including melatonin. As mentioned earlier, melatonin is vital for sleep. It also combats depression, which could affect sleep quality.

It works like this: exposure to sunlight during the day boosts 'dim light melatonin production' which begins after sunset. Spending time in the sun prepares your body for peaceful sleep by boosting din-light melatonin production.

This one of the simplest sleep hacks you can use – and it's completely free! It's as easy as a walk in the park during lunch break, or having a smoothie at an outdoor café. No matter how busy your day, there are still many opportunities to grab some sin.

How much time should you spend in the sun? Ideally, 15 – 20 minutes a day at least. Of course, this also depends on several factors, such as the climate you live in, the season, the time of day, how sensitive your skin is, and how much of your skin is exposed.

Studies show that sitting near a well-lit window is another way to expose your skin to blue light during the daytime. This is the perfect hack for rainy days or when it's too cold to go outside.

Use a Light Therapy Box

If it is difficult for you to get into the sun on a regular basis, a light therapy box is a good alternative. This is a device that emits blue wavelength light. It is designed to balance your circadian rhythm. in the same way that exposure to sunlight does.

Place the box a few feet away from you but do not face it directly. Placing in your peripheral vision is recommended. Expose yourself to the light for 15-30 minutes. Expose as much skin as possible during your session. Ideally, you should do this at the same time every day to maintain your circadian rhythm.

There you go. Another super easy and effortless sleep hack!

CHAPTER 5

SLEEP-FRIENDLY FOOD HACKS

We all love food, and luckily, this food hack includes foods that everybody enjoys. This hack allows you to get creative and prepare dishes that are not only delicious but will also help you sleep like a baby!

The following is a list of sleep-friendly foods that have been proven to be highly beneficial for sleep. Incorporate them into your diet, especially at dinnertime and be amazed at how the quality of your sleep improves.

- Kiwi
- Fatty fish (salmon, tuna, halibut, mackerel)
- Cherries
- Poultry
- Avocadoes
- Leafy greens, especially spinach

- Nuts, especially pistachios, almonds, and walnuts
- Cheese
- Chamomile tea
- Starchy foods (potatoes, yams, plantains)
- Peanut butter
- Bananas
- Oatmeal and cereal

These foods contain tryptophan, an amino acid that produces serotonin (a hormone the relieves stress, promotes calmness and uplifts the mood). They also contain the all-important melatonin. Eating these foods regularly promotes what scientists call "sleep hygiene". Sleep hygiene means the food habits that we develop, especially before bedtime, to promote sleep.

Best of all, the foods above are not only well-liked by most people but can be combined in salads, desserts, casseroles or eaten on their own on a daily basis. Make it a habit to eat at least one or two of them at every meal, but especially dinnertime. A handful of nuts, a small bowl of oatmeal or a banana make great before-bedtime snacks too.

I think you would agree that practicing food hygiene is one hack that is easy and enjoyable. So, get creative! Play around with sleep-friendly foods and see which ones make the best sleep hacks for your body.

Don't sabotage your sleep by indulging in the following foods:

o   Coffee, soda and energy drinks, which are all high in caffeine (even non-cola soda contains caffeine)

o   Chocolate

o   Spicy foods and chili

o   Peppermint

o   Alcohol (alcohol may make you drowsy for a while but in fact, it is a big sleep disrupter. Alcoholic beverages will make it difficult for your brain to enter into the deep sleep cycle necessary for quality sleep)

o   High-fat foods

o   Salty foods.

o   Foods high in water content such as watermelon and cantaloupe. You want to avoid disrupting your sleep with frequent trips to the bathroom!

This is not to say that you must cut these foods out of your diet permanently. Personally, I wouldn't be able to function without my morning cup of coffee. Just try to limit them to daytime hours in order to prep your body for a good night's sleep.

If you must have that hamburger or bag of chips, have it for lunch. Make it a rule to abstain from sleep-disrupting foods from noon onwards.

CHAPTER 6

ACUPRESSURE MAT HACK

This a regular mat padded with foam and covered in sacking. It is embedded with plastic disks that have protruding spikes. It is believed that these mats are an adaptation of the bed of nails used by yogis during meditation – ouch! But don't worry; an acupressure mat is nowhere near as hard! It's similar to a massage chair or an acupressure machine but at a fraction of the cost.

Prices range from $20 to $40and they are available online. Acupressure mats are surprisingly durable and easily washable as well.

How does an acupressure mat work?

❑ A typical mat contains more than 800 "massage points" or spikes that deeply massage your body. They relax tense muscles, relieve aches and pains and promote great sleep.

28

❏ Millions of people who have used them report an immediate improvement in sleep quality, especially when they use them in the evenings.

❏ An acupressure mat also works like a charm to relieve back, neck and joint pain. If you suffer from these conditions in addition to sleep deprivation, you are getting a double benefit.

❏ It improves metabolism and digestion so it is really a "holistic hack" for overall health and wellbeing.

❏ It improves blood circulation, which also promotes sound sleep.

How to use an acupressure mat

The mat is very versatile and can be used on chairs, benches, your bed or the floor. It's light enough to carry to the beach or the park. All you have to do is lie on it for a minimum of 2o to 30 minutes daily, or for as long as you want to. You can use it twice daily if you have the time, once in the morning and then in the evening. It is perfectly safe and has no side effects.

❏ Schedule time daily to enjoy a relaxing session – just as you would with a massage therapist.

❑ The first 3 – 5 minutes will be painful but as you settle in, you will get comfortable and enjoy the sensation. It has been described by users as "pure bliss".

❑ For an intense massage, it's best to use it on the floor. Some people thoroughly enjoy it but others find it too uncomfortable., Experiment with different surfaces and see which one works best for you.

❑ The more skin that is exposed against the mat, the greater the benefit. You might want to wear a bathing suit or even go completely nude if you are assured of privacy.

❑ If you are into yoga or meditation, you can practice on the mat for added stress relief and relaxation.

Restrictions

There are generally no restrictions on gender or even age. There are only three exceptions:

❑ If you are pregnant

❑ If you are suffering from skin rashes

❑ If you have cuts, wounds or burns on your skin.

CHAPTER 7

BINAURAL BEATS AND MUSIC THERAPY

Binaural beats are auditory tones that affect brainwaves. The frequency of the beats changes the brainwaves to achieve specific outcomes. Binaural beats are used to improve creativity, concentration, and sleep.

How do binaural beats work?

➢ The sound frequencies presented to each ear are different, therefore, a good set of stereo headphones is required. There are special binaural beat headphones available on the marketplace but any good quality headphones will work just as well.

➢ The frequency of each tone must be less than 30 Hz to be effective. This allows the two different beats to be heard together as a single tone.

➤ The brain interprets the two beats as one consistent sound frequency. This is called the Frequency Following Response. It then regulates its waves in accordance with this tone.

➤ Binaural beats are designed with specific algorithms to hack your brain into a certain frequency. Our brains use different frequencies when performing tasks. For example, it uses Delta and Theta waves for sleep. They are related to relaxation, calm and deep sleep. The binaural beat you listen to hacks your brain to generate these brainwaves.

If you are thinking that binaural beats are some kind of weird, alien music, you are totally mistaken. They are amazingly soothing, ethereal and beautiful. You will experience calm, blissful thoughts as you gently drift off to sleep.

If you enjoy it, you can invest in an audio track package or a subscription, which is very affordable. Just remember that you need a really good set of headphones to really benefit from this hack.

Music therapy

If nature sounds or binaural beats just aren't your thing, there is another alternative. If you love music then music therapy is the perfect hack for you. Music therapy or the use of soothing music has been scientifically proven to promote relaxation and sleep. It is a great alleviator of physical stress which could be causing bad sleep. Moreover, music therapy has been shown to balance the circadian rhythm.

How does it work?

When soothing waves of music interconnect with our brainwaves, we begin to relax and drift off to sleep. Over time, the brain will associate this type of music with restfulness and sleep. It will learn to relax almost immediately and you will have no trouble falling asleep.

What is meant by "soothing" music?

Loud, fast music like hard rock or rap will alert your brain and keep you awake. Soothing music is the opposite. It is slower with soft beats and rhythms. Research has shown that the best music for sleep is:

➢ **Classical music like Sonatas and piano pieces**. A popular favorite is Beethoven's Moonlight Sonata

➢ **Soft rock**. If you're a rock lover, save the hard rock for daytime. Instead, listen to your favorite soft rock tracks during bedtime. These should be tracks where the emphasis is on melody and words rather than on beat.

➢ **Ambient music**. This includes instrumentals with slow to medium beats. You can find instrumental versions of your favorite songs as well. One of the most popular is Hotel California.

➢ **Hymns**. A great choice for the more religious or spiritually-inclined.

Again, it's a good idea to experiment with these different audio therapies as well. You may find that some genres – not necessarily your favorite – work better for you. Who knows? You may not be religious but discover that hymns do the trick for you!

CHAPTER 8

AROMATHERAPY

A lot of people look at aromatherapy with skepticism. They see it as a fad or something used by meditation and spiritual fanatics.

But science has shown that the scent of essential oils affects our brain in various ways. They can calm anxiety, uplift mood and inspire optimism. Most importantly, they are potent insomnia-busters.

How to use essential oils

Using a diffuser. The best way to use essential oils is to inhale the scent. This is because the olfactory nerves in our nose are directly connected to the brain. The scent of the essential oil travels quickly to the brain, triggering sleep-promoting hormones. You also get the added bonus of your room and home being filled with the beautiful fragrance.

A diffuser is very inexpensive and can be bought almost anywhere essential oils are sold. A cotton ball dipped in essential oil and placed near your bedside is a good alternative as well.

Essential oils are 100% safe to use when diffused. Children and pets will not be harmed by inhaling the scent. In fact, your kids, cars, and dogs will enjoy better quality sleep too!

Use essential oils in the bath. A few drops of essential oil in a warm bath creates a blissful and relaxing experience. The warm water and the scent of the oil will work together to put you in the perfect mood for sleep.

Note: Take warm baths an hour before bedtime and not right before. Warm water boosts circulation for a while, which will keep you awake.

Spray bed linen with essential oil. Use a spray bottle to lightly spray your bedsheets and pillowcases. Thus will create a fragrant sleep haven that will last all night.

To follow is a list of essential oils recommended for sleep problems.

❑ **Chamomile essential oil.** This is a natural sedative extremely inductive to sleep.

❑ **Marjoram essential oil.** A natural antidepressant and anxiety reliever that aids in better sleep.

❑ **Clary Sage essential oil.** This is also a very calming and natural sedative.

❑ **Frankincense essential oil.** This is hailed as a miracle oil because of its many therapeutic properties. As a sleep agent, it lowers your body temperature to the optimum level required for quality sleep. It also clears the nasal passages, allowing you to breathe deeply during sleep.

❑ **Ylang Ylang essential oil.** Lowers blood pressure and stimulates feelings of tranquility and peacefulness.

❑ **Lavender essential oil.** This oil has been used for centuries for calmness and relaxation. In addition to its heavenly scent, lavender is a great sleep agent. It promotes REM sleep. This is a deep sleep during which the heartbeat slows down and muscles relax completely. This is the best quality of sleep you can get.

❑ **Orange and rose essential oils.** When combined together, these two oils make a potent, blissfully fragrant sedative.

❑ **Valerian essential oil.** The scent of this oil will help you stay sound asleep all night. It also relaxes the body and promotes a sense of tranquility and wellbeing.

❑ **Bergamot essential oil.** Promotes better sleep by lowering heart rate and blood pressure. It also gives you the added benefit of relieving anxiety.

On the other end of the spectrum are oils that promote energy and alertness. Some of these include rosemary, peppermint, grapefruit, lemon, and cypress. Products containing these ingredients may also chase away sleep, so avoid using them in the evening. Instead of relaxing you, they will give you a big energy boost. However, they are great hacks to use during the morning, especially on hectic days when you start feeling drained.

CHAPTER 9

HELPFUL SLEEP TIPS

The following are additional biohacking tips that just make sense. In fact, you might be using them already. In addition to the more specific hacks discussed here, these extra little tweaks will give you added benefit.

Regular exercise. Having a regular exercise routine improves overall health and a healthy body plays a big role in quality sleep. Exercise does not have to be an aerobics class or a gym workout. Biking, swimming and nature walks are equally healthy. Just make sure you are exercising your body regularly.

Remember, exercising before bedtime is not a good idea as it will energize you.

Unwind before bedtime. Spend an hour in a relaxing activity before going to bed. Read a book, meditate if you're into it, or spend time in quiet conversation with your partner.

Avoid stressful activities that will keep you up for hours. If you're high-strung, or easily scared, do not watch horror movies. Do not start arguing with your spouse about finances. Avoid getting into any situation that could cause you stress.

Quiet surroundings encourage sound sleep. If family members are up and about, ask them to keep noise to a minimum. Turn off your cell phone if possible. Fix any noisy devices like air conditioners or clanking boilers.

Take stock of any additional noises that could disrupt sleep. If you are a light sleeper this is doubly important.

A good way to tune out noise is by playing soft music or nature sounds in your bedroom throughout the night.

Buy the best quality essential oils. Not all essential oils are created equal. For optimum benefit, buy only the best quality. These should be labeled 100% pure or 1oo% organic.

Invest in a top-quality mattress. Your mattress is not something you want to skimp on. It is the "foundation" that will make biohacking truly optimal.

You may not know this, but most mattresses are padded with highly toxic materials. Flame retardants especially are extremely harmful to health as well as quality sleep. These toxins may take years to air out and in the meantime, you are breathing them in!

A 1oo% natural or organic mattress is one of the soundest investments you can make. Do your due diligence and take time to shop around and look at various brands. It will be expensive but look at it this way: don't you value your health more?

Switch of the Wi-Fi. Wi-Fi waves can interfere with your brain waves during sleep. Simply switch it off and generally, do not keep any routers in your bedroom.

Make sure your bedroom temperature is right for sleep. The best temperature for optimal sleep is 60-67 F. As you fall asleep, your body temperature drops, so keeping your room cool will aid this process. Maintain your room at this temperature as much as possible, Try wearing socks and prepare a hot water bottle when you are cold.

Take supplements that promote sleep. Natural supplements are totally different from sleeping pills as they are totally natural and have no side effects. They may be helpful hacks if your body is lacking certain sleep- promoting vitamins and minerals. Vitamin B-5, vitamin B- 12, vitamin D and magnesium, iron, calcium, and Vitamin E are important for stabilizing the circadian rhythm. You can buy them over the counter supplements to improve your sleep.

CHAPTER 10

PUTTING IT ALL TOGETHER

So, what can we take away from all this?

❑ We've seen how we can use biohacking to optimize sleep.

❑ We've seen that hacking sleep does not require advanced scientific knowledge or complex gadgets.

❑ Biohacking is a series of small lifestyle changes that optimize how your body functions.

❑ Biohacking is hassle-free and costs almost nothing. It is a totally natural way to promote sleep.

So, how do you start to use the biohacks discussed here? Which ones are best to start with? Can we use them all together? How can you put together the perfect biohacking plan?

If you are new to biohacking, it's normal to feel a little overwhelmed. The key is to start small. Think of biohacking as a toolbox. All of the techniques discussed here are the different tools in that toolbox. First, you must customize these tools to meet your needs. Then you need to tweak them to get optimal results.

For example, let's say you want to start with binaural beats. Download a few tracks and use them for a few nights. Record any changes in your sleep and rate them on a scale of 1 to 1o. 1 would be remarkable improvement and 1o would be no improvement.

Next, try listening to music or nature sounds and see if certain tracks give you better sleep. Record and rate your findings. Play with different audio tracks until you settlen on the type of auditory hacks that work best for you. Next, move onto a new tool and repeat the process.

If you choose to use an acupressure mat, try it out on different surfaces and see how it feels. If you find that it's just too uncomfortable, discard it and move on to another hack, and so on.

Remember, there is no best or worst hack for sleep. The golden rule is what works best for you.

Suggestions:

➤ Start with one or two hacks that resonate the most with you. Give yourself a week or two to experiment and see what results you get.

➤ Incorporate the hacks that give you the best sleep into your daily routine. Practice them regularly until they become habits.

➤ Move on to another hack and repeat the process.

➤ I recommend starting with the sleep-friendly food hack. It is the easiest and requires nothing more than consuming the foods listed here.

➤ Practice makes perfect! You may notice immediate results or gradual improvement in your sleep over days or weeks, Don't give up too quickly.

➢ Typically, however, biohacking tools do not always give immediate results. Your brain needs time to adapt to the new triggers you are teaching it. Patience and practice are the key here. Allow two weeks as a timeframe for each hack to start working before moving on to a new one.

Remember: Biohacking is a process of experimentation. It is a process of discovery through trial and error of what works best for your sleep patterns.

CONCLUSION

Sleep deprivation is a problem that can bring your life to a standstill. It can hinder you from functioning at your peak. It can seriously affect your mental and physical health. It can damage relationships. More importantly, it prevents you from enjoying life.

Biohacking has been scientifically proven to improve sleep quality. There is nothing to lose and so much to gain by implementing these hacks into your routine.

Finally, biohacking is fun! Once you get the hang of it, you will want to hack other areas of your life like academic and sports performance, weight loss and even better rapport with others. With biohacking, the sky is truly the limit.

Printed by Libri Plureos GmbH in Hamburg,
Germany